Your Amazing Itty Bitty™ Healthy Habits Book

15 Steps to Embrace Your New Way of Life

Dr. Mary Zennett

Published by Itty Bitty™ Publishing
A subsidiary of S & P Productions, Inc.

Printed in the United States of America

Itty Bitty Publishing
311 Main Street, Suite D
El Segundo, CA 90245
(310) 640-8885

ISBN: 978-1-950326-98-3

Dedication

For my dear mom, Frances, who taught me the foundations of good health and who had such a heart to make the world a better place.

Stop by our Itty Bitty™ website to find interesting blog entries regarding healthy lifestyle habits.

www.IttyBittyPublishing.com

Or visit Dr. Mary Zennett at

https://movementforglobalhealth.com/

Table of Contents

Introduction

Introduction

Natural health advocates have made tremendous strides in raising public awareness about safe product selections. Chemical-free, fragrance-free, toxin-free products all reduce risk of illness, enhance longevity, and improve quality of life.

Yet so many people still don't know enough about natural health. Less costly options are still preferred, which need to change if we are going to survive as a species.

Our soil is depleted of nutrients and abounds with pesticides. Products that we use on our face and spray on our carpets are full of chemicals that can hurt or even kill us.

This book is written to inform, educate, and activate. It serves as a "driver's manual" for consumers. Select healthy products, reap the rewards. Share with others. The only way to offset massive commercial influence to consume unsafe products is to change one person at a time. And to share knowledge with friends and family.

Together we will create a healthy world.

Step 1
See the Truth Uncovered

Did you know the U.S. ranks last in health quality among all industrialized countries? (1)

1. Our planet is ailing. The same toxins that are destroying our world are destroying our health. Our healthcare system doesn't disclose the effect of toxins in our air, food, and water in maintaining health and preventing illness.

2. Dr. Zach Bush, a specialist in endocrinology and internal medicine says, "Over the last 25 years we have seen the most profound explosion of chronic disease in human history, which suggests that environmental factors now contribute to genetic, neurologic, auto-immune, and metabolic injuries that underpin the collapse of health in children and adults." (2)

3. Problems once considered solved are back with a vengeance. Did you know more than 500,000 children have detectable levels of lead in their blood? In this day and age, children exposed to potent neurotoxins such as lead definitely need our attention!

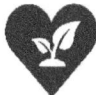

Time to Face the Facts

"The United States is among the wealthiest nations in the world, but it is far from the healthiest. Americans live shorter lives and experience more injuries and illnesses than people in other high-income countries." (3)

- Popular food choices are often alarmingly unhealthy, even toxic. Yet they are marketed to whet your appetites and tantalize your taste buds. Examples are fast food and processed foods.
- U.S. water is considered safe, but a new study reveals that "tap water exposure to carcinogenic contaminants corresponds to 105,887 estimated lifetime cancer cases." (4)
- We must step outside our comfort zones, learn, and act. It is said that lifestyle changes will reverse the course of chronic disease by up to 85%. Make up your mind not to be a casualty!

We are here pioneering a new way of life. We are up against massive obstacles, but with forethought and daily action steps we can rise, overcome, and thrive! In fact, our survival as individuals and as a planet depends on it. Let's dive in.

Step 2
Let Your Food Be Your Medicine

What you put in your mouth is one of the largest determinants of your quality of life long-term.

1. You know junk food is bad, but how do you resist the urges and cravings? One of the first steps is to research and plan your meals in advance. When you shop, resist the urge to buy junk food and look for healthy snack options. Read labels, eat regularly, and keep healthy snacks on hand. Drink plenty of water, especially before meals, which reduces cravings.
2. Know your food weaknesses. When tempted by fast food, have a small snack on hand so you can take a pass on fast food. Celebrate driving past the drive-thru!
3. Teach your kids early about healthy foods. Today, many food selections for children are literally toxic. A link is suspected between junk food and ADHD, autism, and possibly cancer.

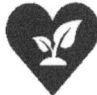

Take a Foodie Deep-Dive

- Treat yourself to some healthy diet investigative work. Go online or to a favorite bookstore and explore healthy recipe books for main courses and snacks. Look for books by certified health coaches or nutritionists who are aware of current food trends.
- Consider joining a Meetup focused on healthy eating; you'll meet some wonderful people and exchange great ideas. Connecting with other empowered people is both inspiring and motivating.
- Embrace the three-step process of change:

    - Learn
    - Take action
    - Share

Learn: Find new foods and ways to prepare them.

Take action: Shop for healthy foods and practice cooking new recipes.

Share: Enjoy sharing new cuisine creations with family and friends and get in the habit of exchanging good recipes.

Step 3
The Genetically Modified Deception

Since the 1990s, GMOs (genetically modified organisms) have been prevalent in food.

1. According to Greenpeace, what most people don't know is the connection between GMOs and pesticides. (5) The surge of genetically engineered crops is one of the main drivers of increased use of chemicals and pesticides in agriculture, which are harmful to people, the environment, and wildlife.
2. GMOs were widely accepted until doctors and scientists realized that people were getting sick from eating GMO foods. In 2009, the American Academy of Environmental Medicine advised that GMOs not be consumed because they had not been properly tested for human consumption, and because there was ample evidence of probable harm. (6)
3. Read and learn about GMOs, the research, and the risks. It can be lifesaving! Find out more at https://www.nongmoproject.org

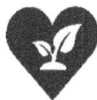

Just Say No to GMOs

Make sure you understand why this is so important.

- Over 80 percent of all GMOs grown worldwide are engineered for herbicide intolerance. As a result, the use of toxic herbicides such as Roundup has increased 15-fold since GMOs were introduced.
- GMO crops are responsible for the emergence of "superbugs" which can only be killed with even more toxic poisons like 2,4-D (a major ingredient in Agent Orange). GMOs are a direct extension of chemical agriculture and are developed and sold by the world's biggest chemical companies.
- Remember, it's ideal to eat organic foods, but eating non-GMO is so much safer than GMO. And if you find a few boxed brands that are non-GMO and organic, support them! The biggest challenge is being surrounded by food choices that look tasty and appetizing, but we can no longer be fooled.

You will want to eat only non-GMO and organic whenever possible!

Step 4
High Fructose Corn Syrup

Leading health expert Dr. Mark Hyman wrote a sobering, must-read article, "5 Reasons High Fructose Corn Syrup Will Kill You." (7)

1. Did you know high fructose corn syrup is used in almost all packaged foods and sodas consumed in America today? Read Dr. Hyman's article and take note of the massive marketing deception of products that contain high fructose corn syrup.
2. Did you know high fructose corn syrup is highly addictive and will make you hungrier? So, avoid the traps. How? Avoid products labeled HFCS (high fructose corn syrup), fructose, fructose syrup, maize syrup, natural corn syrup.
3. You probably know that HFCS is very affordable and has a long shelf life. You realize clever marketing ploys have helped make these HFCS foods very appealing. They may be clever, but you are informed and empowered, and steer clear of all foods containing high fructose corn syrup.

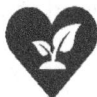

Take This Battle to Heart

When used in moderation, high fructose corn syrup (HFCS) is a major cause of heart disease, obesity, cancer, dementia, liver failure, tooth decay, and more.

Armed with knowledge, you steer clear of foods containing high fructose corn syrup.

- Soda
- Candy
- Bread and crackers
- Canned fruit
- Granola bars
- Cereal
- Salad dressings
- Snack foods
- TV dinners
- Energy drinks
- Applesauce
- Packaged cookies, pastries, cupcakes
- Juice drinks
- Fast foods
- Sauces, including steak sauce
- Ice cream
- Fruit preserves, jams
- Pancake syrup

By reading labels carefully you may find a small number of products listed above that do not contain high fructose corn syrup (HFCS).

Step 5
Beware of Vegetable Oils

Learn the hidden risks!

1. Dr. Jason Fung wrote an alarming article, "The Shocking Origin of Vegetable Oil-Garbage!" (8) He describes the dilemma cotton growers faced with the staggering waste of cotton seeds. Proctor & Gamble had been using cottonseed oil to make candles and soap but learned the oil could be hydrogenated to create trans-fat.
2. Dr. Fung describes the birth of Crisco, which is derived from cottonseed oil, an industrial waste product. He aptly states, "Nobody actually knew whether we should be shoving this former toxic waste into our mouths."
3. Health leaders like Chris Kresser have also raised alarms. "Industrial seed oils were originally used in the soapmaking process. So how did these industrial byproducts end up on our plates?" (9)

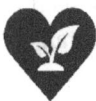

Learn the Why and What: Oils to Avoid

- Did you know vegetable oil is pro-inflammatory? Dr. Cate Shanahan reports these oils are "… high in unstable fatty acids that break down into toxins when you cook with them and when you eat them for years and years." She also advocates that eliminating the high-PUFA (polyunsaturated fatty acids) seed oils is the *single best thing* you can do to help your immune system beat corona-virus. The insanely high level of inflammatory chemicals in our bloodstream, lungs, and other tissues cause metabolic pandemonium. We start drowning in our own fluids and can't oxygenate. (10)
- Are you aware that by Nov. 2013 the FDA removed partially hydrogenated oils from the "generally recognized as safe" list of human foods?
- Avoid these eight vegetable oils named the "Hateful 8" by Dr. Cate Shanahan:

  - Canola
  - Corn
  - Cottonseed
  - Soy
  - Sunflower
  - Safflower
  - Grapeseed
  - Rice bran

Step 6
Genetic Engineering: Don't Mess With Mother Nature!

One topic that is not on our radar (and should be) is the release of genetically engineered microbes into our environment. You read that right, and we owe Jeffrey Smith, founder of the Institute for Responsible Technology for sounding the alarm on this one. With little fanfare, industry is releasing genetically engineered bacteria, viruses, and insects into the world!

1. In Smith's words, "Genetic engineering techniques have become so inexpensive we can easily and permanently reorder the code of life, irreversibly altering wild populations of any organism that contains DNA. (11)
2. In May 2021, the first genetically engineered mosquitos were released in the Florida Keys. Public resistance was strong but could not overcome industry pressure. Public concerns: What if the experiment to kill wild female mosquitos doesn't work? What happens if you're bit by one of these mosquitos?

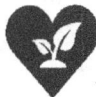

Raise Your Voice to Stop Genetic Engineering!

Are you aware there are no regulations to stop this? The plan is to get past Florida and release these mosquitos all across the U.S. We need public pressure and organized, persistent action.

Become familiar with the Protect Nature Now Coalition and its two goals:

- Stop all outdoor release of genetically engineered microbes.
- Stop all gain of function research in laboratories that would cause pandemics if they escaped. The term *gain of function* refers to the deliberate design of virulent pathogens.

The Protect Nature Now Coalition has grants to run professional campaigns to empower your tribe and reach stakeholders, including legislators. To learn more visit: https://protectnaturenow.com/

Remember Jeffrey Smith's words, "Covid-19 is a glaring example of how microorganisms and viruses, genetically engineered or not, can quickly encircle the globe."

We are all stakeholders here!

Step 7
Water: It's Your Life

Water is essential for life to exist. All living organisms use water to take in substances that generate energy and flush out toxins and waste products.

1. About 75% of the earth is water but less than 2.5% is freshwater, and only 31% of that is available for use. This means less than 1% of the earth's water is available for use. Water is a very precious resource!
2. According to a 2008 WHO (World Health Organization) report on drinkable water and sanitation, about 885 million people (one-eighth of the world's population) have no access to safe water. About 3.6 million people die annually from diseases resulting from unsafe drinking water. (12)
3. In many countries today, the biggest source of water pollution is agriculture - not cities or industries.

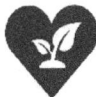

Water Alert!

- According to Environmental Working Group (EWG), "The regulatory system meant to ensure the safety of America's drinking water is broken. There are no legal limits for more than 160 unregulated contaminants in U.S. tap water. For some other chemicals, the EPA's maximum contaminant levels, or MCLs, haven't been updated in almost 50 years." (13)
- You must check the safety of your tap water. Visit https://ewg.org/tapwater/ for analysis of contaminants in your local water supply, potential health risks, and water filtration that can protect your home.

Take some time to learn the history of clean water in your region. What action steps can you take to support clean water in your community? What organizations can you align with? Review EWG's article, "7 Questions to Ask Your Elected Officials About Tap Water" (14) and find a way to meet with legislators in person or on Zoom.

To learn more about home water filtration systems read this guide by Environmental Working Group:
https://www.ewg.org/tapwater/water-filter-guide.php

Step 8
Do a Deep Clean of Your Cleaning Products

How *clean* are your cleaning products?

1. Did you know household cleaning products have contained toxins for many decades, unbeknownst to consumers focused on keeping their homes clean?
2. Did you know the U.S. government currently allows over 40,000 chemicals in consumer products, and the vast majority have not been tested for safety?
3. Environmental Working Group reveals that 53% of cleaning products contain ingredients known to harm the lungs.

Are you aware that some cleaning products have tested to be carcinogenic, hormone disrupting, and neurotoxic?

These risks impact the person using the cleaners, as well as everyone in the home who may suffer the aftereffects.

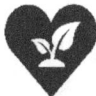

Cleveland Clinic's Important Warning:
Potentially Dangerous Chemicals Exist in Every Room of Your Home

Resources are available for help:

- Environmental Working Group's "Guide to Healthy Cleaning" (15) is very comprehensive. For 14 months, EWG scientists worked diligently, analyzing product labels, technical documents, government and academic toxicity databases, and more to compile this very thorough guide.
- Organic Consumer's Association has published a very detailed, hands-on resource for cleaning dos and don'ts. (16) It provides invaluable information to help keep you and your household safe.
- Listen carefully to EWG when they tell you to avoid the following products altogether:

    - Air fresheners
    - Antibacterial products
    - Fabric softeners and dryer sheets
    - Drain and oven cleaners

Action Step: Take out all the products from under your sink and read the product labels to see which ones you feel safe with. Use EWG's resources as a guide to help you.

Step 9
Beauty Inside and Out

Would you know if your beauty products contain toxins? Would you believe more than 40 countries have banned 1,400 chemicals in cosmetic products, compared with only nine in the US?

1. How does it make you feel to know that it is perfectly legal for companies to use ingredients linked to cancer, endocrine disruption, and reproductive harm in the cosmetics and personal care products we use every day?

2. From the *Global Journal of Medical Research,* "The use of cosmetic products is increasing around the world and a variety of chemical compounds used in the manufacture of these products grows at the same time. In this way, the risk of intoxication, allergic processes, prolonged chemical exposure, side effects, and indiscriminate use are also increased. (17) The authors point to an emerging public health crisis with the indiscriminate use of cosmetics.

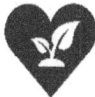

Do Your Research Carefully

Use the Skin-Deep database to look up every cosmetic and hair product you consider using. (18)

- With 80,000 products rated for safety, you will learn valuable information. Try to use EWG-verified products that Environmental Working Group rates high for safety.
- Please share this important information with your family and friends. Cosmetics are so popular and so fashionable, yet not enough people are talking about potentially serious health risks when using toxic ingredients on our skin. There are healthier cosmetic options! Think about the number of fashion-savvy consumers of all ages who are completely uninformed on this issue—it's massive!
- As a group, we need to get the word out. Think of how many people you know who love their cosmetics and look wonderful! Chances are they have absolutely no idea of the risk of ingredients in many cosmetics. You'll be doing them a huge favor by letting them know. Also, let them know that the complexity of chemicals poses greater risks to the environment as well.

Be aware—take action and share!

Step 10
Saving Our Soil

Our land has nourished the world since the beginning of time. Industrialized agricultural practices have damaged the landscape so severely there are legitimate concerns that there will be no topsoil left to grow crops within 60 years.

1. Did you know the boom in global agricultural productivity that followed WWII was achieved in large part through the intensive use of pesticides and chemical fertilizers?
2. Are you aware that agricultural practices like heavy tilling, heavy chemicals, overgrazing, and CAFO (concentrated animal feeding operation) have done extensive global damage to the soil?
3. What do you think about Chris Kresser's statement that the farming system needs a complete overhaul? Kresser states, "We're overfed and undernourished" from eating food grown in depleted soils. (19)

Food for thought: How might depleted soils be impacting the nutrient levels in your food today?

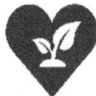

Learn to Love Our Soil Again

- Chris Kresser continues: "When animals and agriculture are integrated, a sustainable farm can be net carbon positive, meaning it returns carbon to the soil instead of releasing it into the air. The answer to climate change isn't veganism or lab-grown meat; instead, the answer lies in sustainable farms where crops, animals, and soil are integrated for mutual benefits.
- To learn more visit: https://kisstheground.com and become a soil advocate. You'll learn about regenerative organic agriculture and gain a deeper appreciation of the essence of soil and its role in nourishing humanity.
- Get involved! Our soil crisis is an urgent one that needs a lot of us to get involved. Support regenerative farming; you can visit a local farm, learn about it, and support it with your purchases and word-of-mouth referrals.
  https://regenerationinternational.org/

Let farmers know, too. So many farmers are hurting economically right now. Many want to stop using pesticides but don't know where to begin. Introduce them to www.savory.global and https://rodaleinstitute.org for support.

Step 11
The Plight of Plastics

"We're doomed to live with yesterday's plastic pollution, and we are exacerbating the situation with each day of unchanged behavior." Rolf Halden, PhD (20)

1. Did you know the risks of plastics to our health and the environment are massive? Most plastics fragment into smaller particles, which have "profound detrimental consequences for ecosystems, biota, and the environment, but also for the economy and human health?" (21) In the U.S., the average person produces a half-pound of plastic waste every day.
2. Direct health effects that you need to know about include direct toxicity, as in cases of lead, cadmium, mercury, cancer, birth defects, weakened immune systems, hormonal imbalances, and developmental problems in children.
3. Be aware that you are also exposed long-term to massive plastic pollution in the soil and waterways.

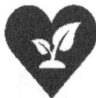

We Must Each Do Our Part

We can be intentional about doing our part to reverse the perilous trends of plastics in our lives.

- Buy food in glass or metal containers; avoid polycarbonate drinking bottles with bisphenol A.
- Do not give young children plastic toys.
- Avoid all PVC (polyvinyl chloride) and styrene products. Stay vigilant for increased use of biodegradable plastics which are in development and on the horizon.
- Learn what initiatives are going on in your community to minimize plastic use and help clean your local water supply.
- Support Ocean Cleanup, whose mission, according to founder Boyan Slat, is to rid the world's oceans of plastic. Every year, millions of tons of plastic enter the oceans, primarily from rivers. As Slat states, this plastic doesn't disappear by itself. Through persistence and advanced technology, waters are getting cleaned up—rivers and oceans! Check out the latest at https://theoceancleanup.com

Consumers play *the most important role* in the plastics equation, with careful use and safe disposal.

Step 12
Moving Past Covid

The Covid pandemic has done more to disrupt life on this planet than anything in recent memory. It's time for us to look beneath the surface to appreciate the full scope of the crisis with an eye on solutions.

1. Did you know hunger is the greatest impact of Covid and also the least talked about? Did you know millions are bordering on starvation around the globe from disrupted supply lines and critical shortages, all fueled by Covid?
2. Locally and globally the most important defense you have against Covid is taking optimal care of your health. We do not hear enough about this. Without nutrient-rich food, you cannot prevent Covid or recover from it.
3. Hippocrates, the father of medicine, did a very thorough examination of all his patients. He even included an assessment of the very ground the person was living on! While that is unheard of today, it drives home the need to discern and appreciate how our food is grown and why it matters.

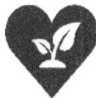

Beat or Avoid Covid: Healthy Immune System and Anti-Inflammatory Diet

- Add vitamins C and D, quercetin, zinc, and glutathione to your daily regimen. Find online doctors who share dosing details. Also, enhance your daily fitness basics with walking and stretching.
- Keep this in mind: these recommendations are for both the vaccinated and unvaccinated. Do not be complacent because you were vaccinated; you can still get Covid and spread it to others. So, take optimal care of your health by eating right and living well.
- Reach out to neighbors locally and globally. Donate to global nonprofits that provide clean food and water to people around the world. Even $5-$10 a month helps a lot. Don't forget about food banks, which have become a lifeline for many. Donate nutrient rich foods, such as canned chicken and fish, unsalted nuts, seeds, and their butters, dry beans, quinoa, honey, chicken, beef, and vegetable broths, and coconut milk. Donate canned items, preferably organic: beans (of all types), tomatoes, vegetables, and soups.

Step 13
Sewer Sludge Shock

Never a dull minute. Just when you have a handle on getting healthy, the topic of sewer sludge crosses your radar.

1. Did you know? "Scientific evidence has confirmed that municipal sewage sludge contains hundreds of dangerous pathogens, toxic heavy metals, flame retardants, endocrine disruptors, carcinogens, pharmaceutical drugs, and other hazardous chemicals coming from hospitals and industrial plants." (22)
2. Think about the following. "When San Francisco offered its residents free compost, many were excited to take it. Few gardeners suspected that the 20 tons of free bags labeled 'organic biosolids compost' actually contained sewage sludge from nine California counties. Angry San Franciscans returned the toxic sludge to the city, dumping it at the mayor's office in protest." (23)
3. Sewage sludge is the end product of the treatment process for any human waste, hospital waste, and industrial waste.

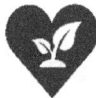

Sewer Sludge: Not Subject to Regulation or Safety Standards

Home gardens, playgrounds, schools, parks, and golf courses can all be legally "fertilized" with bagged sewage sludge, or so-called "fertilizer," without your knowledge.

- Wastewater treatment plants are in the business of cleaning water, not producing clean, non-toxic sludge. The more junk and chemicals they remove from the water, the better job they've done. (24)
- No food crop, aside from USDA organic, is regulated from growing on land treated with sewage sludge "fertilizer."
- Stay active on this issue! Follow the United Sludge-Free Alliance https://usludgefree.org and the Organic Consumers Association (OCA) that hosts a campaign to Stop Toxic Sludge: https://www.organicconsumers.org/campaigns/stop-toxic-sludge

An important article from the guardian reveals: "Companies like Whole Foods, Dole, Heinz and Del Monte won't buy crops grown in biosolids, while Switzerland, the Netherlands and other countries have banned it." (25) The article is an important, sobering reminder of the seriousness of the problems with biosludge.

Step 14
Like Beavers and Ants

Lest we get overwhelmed, consider two of nature's hardest-working members.

1. The ant, through the power of hard work and the support of a large colony, helps create healthy topsoil.
2. Beavers, with remarkable work ethics, are critical to healthy ecosystems. Their dam building improves water quality and provides homes for countless species.
3. Now think about your calling, a purpose you have here on this planet. How, with teammates of like mind and heart, can you help restore the world to greatness? Once you've mastered your own healthy habits it's time to seriously reflect on this. Open your mind and heart to helping create solutions to our world's biggest problems. Many are health-related. Embrace a new era of awakening where we let go of conventional and outdated ways of doing things.

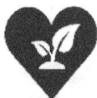

Emulate Humble Leaders With Big Missions

- Dr. Muhammed Yunus is known as the "father of microloans." He helped eradicate dire poverty in Bangladesh, one impoverished worker at a time. (26)
- Dr. G.V. Ramanjaneyulu's mission is to free India of crops grown with pesticides. His organic farming cooperatives give 50-75% back to farmers, compared to conventional markets, which only pay farmers 20-30%. (27)
- Reach deep within yourself and discover how you might dedicate your skills, talents, and passion to creating a healthy world. You've made a tremendous start by fine-tuning your healthy habits and adopting the suggestions in this book. Now reach out to family and friends to share what you have learned. Next, find ways to reach out to people in your community. You will become a resource to help alert others in your community of the risks that exist all around us. As you learn, you will share with others and empower them.
- Like Dr. Yunus, together we will transform the world, one person at a time.

Step 15
Where to Find Resources

1. (1)https://www.commonwealthfund.org/publications/infographic/2014/jun/us-health-care-ranks-last-among-wealthy-countries
2. (2)https://zachbushmd.com/gmo/glyphosate-toxins/
3. (3)https://www.ncbi.nlm.nih.gov/books/NBK154469/
4. (4)https://www.medicalnewstoday.com/articles/326423
5. (5)https://www.greenpeace.org/usa/sustainable-agriculture/issues/gmos/
6. (6)https://www.aaemonline.org/genetically-modified-foods/
7. (7)https://drhyman.com/blog/2011/05/13/5-reasons-high-fructose-corn-syrup-will-kill-you/
8. (8)https://drjasonfung.medium.com/the-shocking-origin-of-vegetable-oil-garbage-1c2ce14ae513 (9)https://chriskresser.com/how-industrial-seed-oils-are-making-us-sick/
9. (10)https://drcate.com/the-hateful-eight-enemy-fats-that-destroy-your-health/
10. (11)https://responsibletechnology.org
11. (12)https://www.who.int/news-room/fact-sheets/detail/drinking-water

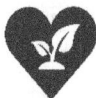

More Resources

- (13)https://www.ewg.org/tapwater/state-of-american-drinking-water.php
- (14)https://www.ewg.org/tapwater/contact-local-government.php
- (15)https://ewg.org/guides/cleaners
- (16)https://organicconsumers.org/hormone-disruptors-everyday-poisons-non-organic-food-body-care-products-water-bottles-and/
- (17)https://globaljournals.org/GJMR_Volume18/6-Cosmetics-and-its-Health-Risks.pdf
- (18)https://www.ewg.org/skindeep/
- (19)https://chriskresser.com/depletion-of-soil-and-what-can-be-done
- (20)https://news.asu.edu/content/asu-researcher-explores-perils-plastics
- (21)https://www.unep.org/news-and-stories/story/plastic-planet-how-tiny-plastic-particles-are-polluting-our-soil
- (22)https://organicconsumers.org/campaigns/stop-toxic-sludge
- (23)https://organicconsumers.org/article_20350/
- (24)https://usludgefree.org/actions-to-do
- (25)https://www.theguardian.com/environment/2019/oct/05/biosolids-toxic-chemicals-pollution
- 26)https://www.nobelprize.org/prizes/peace/2006/yunus/diploma/
- (27)https://csaindia.org/team/ramanjaneyulu-gv/

You've finished. Before you go ...

Post/Share that you finished this book.

Please star rate this book.

Reviews are solid gold to writers. Please take a few minutes to give us some itty bitty feedback.

ABOUT THE AUTHOR

Dr. Mary Zennett® is a loving mom and doctor of 35 years, with a heart for humanity. She is board certified in adult/child and adolescent psychiatry, with advanced training in life-style medicine. Dr. Mary has served as a community psychiatrist for decades. She is passionate about helping the people of the world with quality nutrition and healthy lifestyle habits.

Dr. Mary is the Founder of Movement For Global Health which provides health education and spotlights global leaders in health and the nonprofit Global Health and Heart.

Dr. Mary hosts a podcast, on CTR Media Network https://www.ctrmedianetwork.com/show/movement-for-global-health/ which can be found on YouTube. She features innovative practitioners in the healing arts and invites you to join her.

You can reach Dr. Mary at: drmaryzennett@hushmail.com or through her website https://movementforglobalhealth.com

Together we can create a healthy world!

If you enjoyed this Itty Bitty™ book you might also like …

- **Your Amazing Itty Bitty™ Awaken the Leader Within Book** – Natalie Clayton

- **Your Amazing Itty Bitty™ Self-Care Book** – Denise Schickel

- **Your Amazing Itty Bitty™ Aging Well Book** – Michele McHenry

Or any of the many Amazing Itty Bitty™ books available online at www.ittybittypublishing.com

www.ingramcontent.com/pod-product-compliance
Lightning Source LLC
Chambersburg PA
CBHW060659280326
41933CB00012B/2247